Plant-Based Cooking Made Easy

How To Make Delicious Vegetarian Meals With Quick & Easy Recipes

Brigitte S. Romeo

Plant-Based Cooking Made Easy

© **Copyright 2021 - All rights reserved.**

The content contained within this book may not be reproduced, duplicated or transmitted without direct written permission from the author or the publisher.

Under no circumstances will any blame or legal responsibility be held against the publisher, or author, for any damages, reparation, or monetary loss due to the information contained within this book. Either directly or indirectly.

Legal Notice:

This book is copyright protected. This book is only for personal use. You cannot amend, distribute, sell, use, quote or paraphrase any part, or the content within this book, without the consent of the author or publisher.

Disclaimer Notice:

Please note the information contained within this document is for educational and entertainment purposes only. All effort has been executed to present accurate, up to date, and reliable, complete information. No warranties of any kind are declared or implied. Readers acknowledge that the author is not engaging in the rendering of legal, financial, medical or professional advice. The content within this book has been derived from various sources. Please consult a licensed professional before attempting any techniques outlined in this book.

By reading this document, the reader agrees that under no circumstances is the author responsible for any losses, direct or indirect, which are incurred as a result of the use of information contained within this document, including, but not limited to, errors, omissions, or inaccuracies.

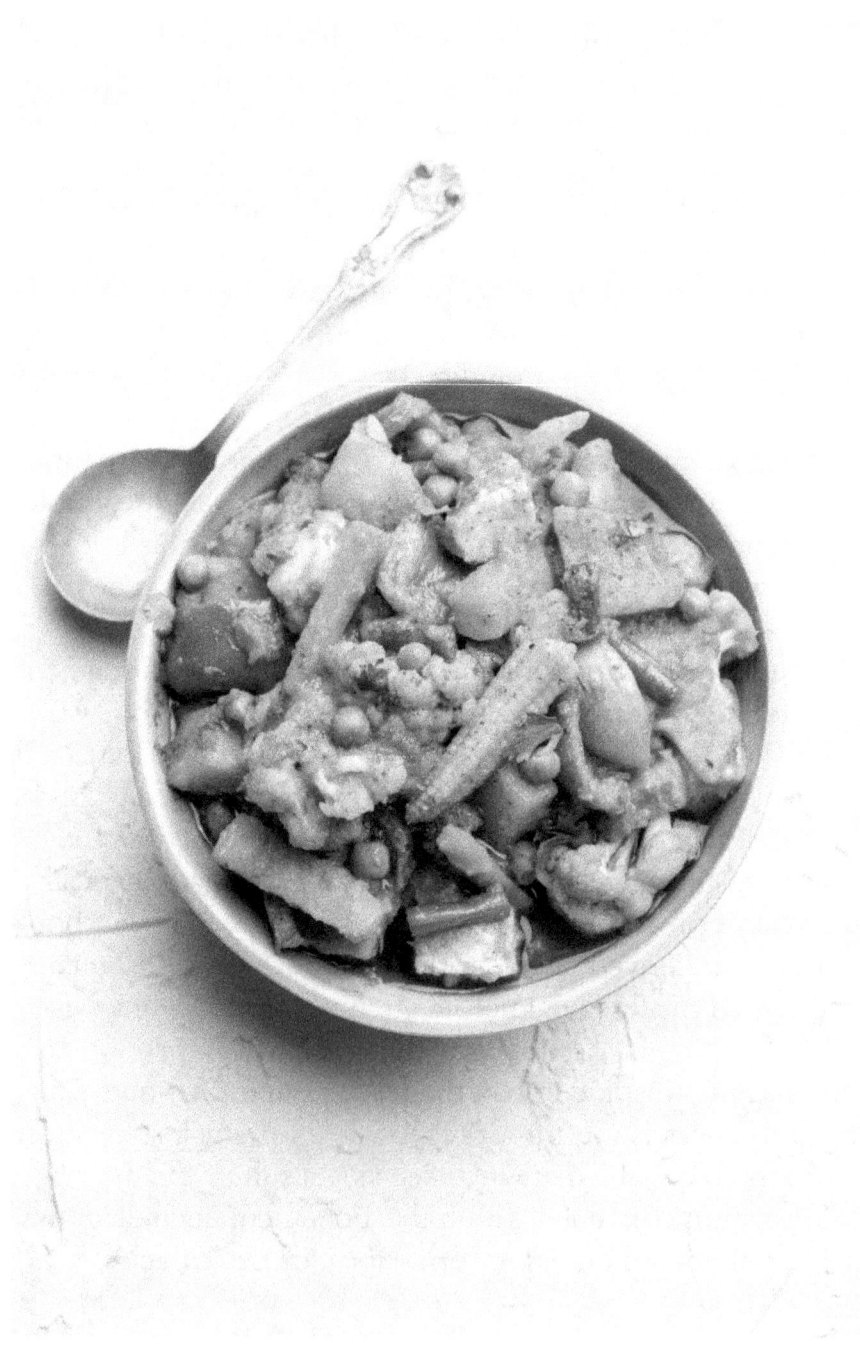

TABLE OF CONTENTS

INTRODUCTION 8

CHAPTER 1: BREAKFAST RECIPES 12

1. Stewed Collard Greens 12
2. Green Beans, Four Ways 15
3. Maple-Glazed Carrots 18
4. Beets, Two Ways 20
5. Crust less Spinach Quiche 23
6. Blueberry-Coconut Quinoa 25
7. Apple-Cinnamon Oatmeal 27

CHAPTER 2: LUNCH RECIPES 30

8. Mexican Beans 31
9. Lime-Mint Soup 33
10. Lemony Kale Salad 34

CHAPTER 3: MAIN MEALS RECIPES 36

11. Moroccan Chickpea Rolls 37
12. Smoky Cajun Bowl 39
13. Sloppy Cajun Burgers 41

CHAPTER 4: VEGETABLES, SALADS AND SIDES RECIPES 44

14. Garlic Roasted Carrots 44
15. Baked Parmesan Mushrooms 46
16. Buttery Garlic Green Beans 48
17. Roasted Butternut Squash Puree 50
18. Irish Bombay Potatoes 52
19. Healthy Mashed Sweet Potato 54
20. Spinach Tomato Quesadilla 56

21. LENTIL TACOS 58

CHAPTER 5: DESSERT RECIPES 60

22. CARDAMOM DATE BITES 60
23. SWEET POTATO PIE NICE CREAM 62
24. PEANUT BUTTER NICE CREAM 64
25. NO BAKE APPLE PIE 65
26. CASHEW-CHOCOLATE TRUFFLES 66
27. CRUSTY ROSEMARY BREAD 68
28. CHEWY OLIVE PARMESAN BREAD 71

CHAPTER 6: SNACK RECIPES 74

29. BAKED POTATOES WITH AVOCADO PICO DE GALLO 74
30. FLOURLESS DARK CHOCOLATE CAKE 76
31. CREAMY PEACH ICE POPS 79
32. MELON-LIME SORBET 81
33. MANDARIN AMBROSIA 83
34. COCONUT-QUINOA PUDDING 84
35. STUFFED PEARS WITH HAZELNUTS 86

CHAPTER 7: JUICES AND SMOOTHIES RECIPES 88

36. HEALTHY PURPLE SMOOTHIE 88
37. MOM'S FAVOURITE KALE SMOOTHIE 90
38. CREAMY GREEN SMOOTHIE 91
39. STRAWBERRY AND ARUGULA SMOOTHIE 92
40. EMMA'S AMAZING SMOOTHIE 93
41. GOOD-TO-GO MORNING SMOOTHIE 94

CHAPTER 8: OTHER RECIPES 96

42. SPINACH & ORANGE SALAD 97
43. LIME-MACERATED MANGOS 98

44.	RASPBERRY CHIA PUDDING	100
45.	LEMON MOUSSE	101
46.	BANANA MANGO ICE CREAM	102
47.	RASPBERRY CHIA PUDDING SHOTS	103
48.	SAUTÉED BOSC PEARS WITH WALNUTS	104
49.	MANGO & PAPAYA AFTER-CHOP	105
50.	GREEK-STYLE GARBANZO BEANS	106

CONCLUSION **108**

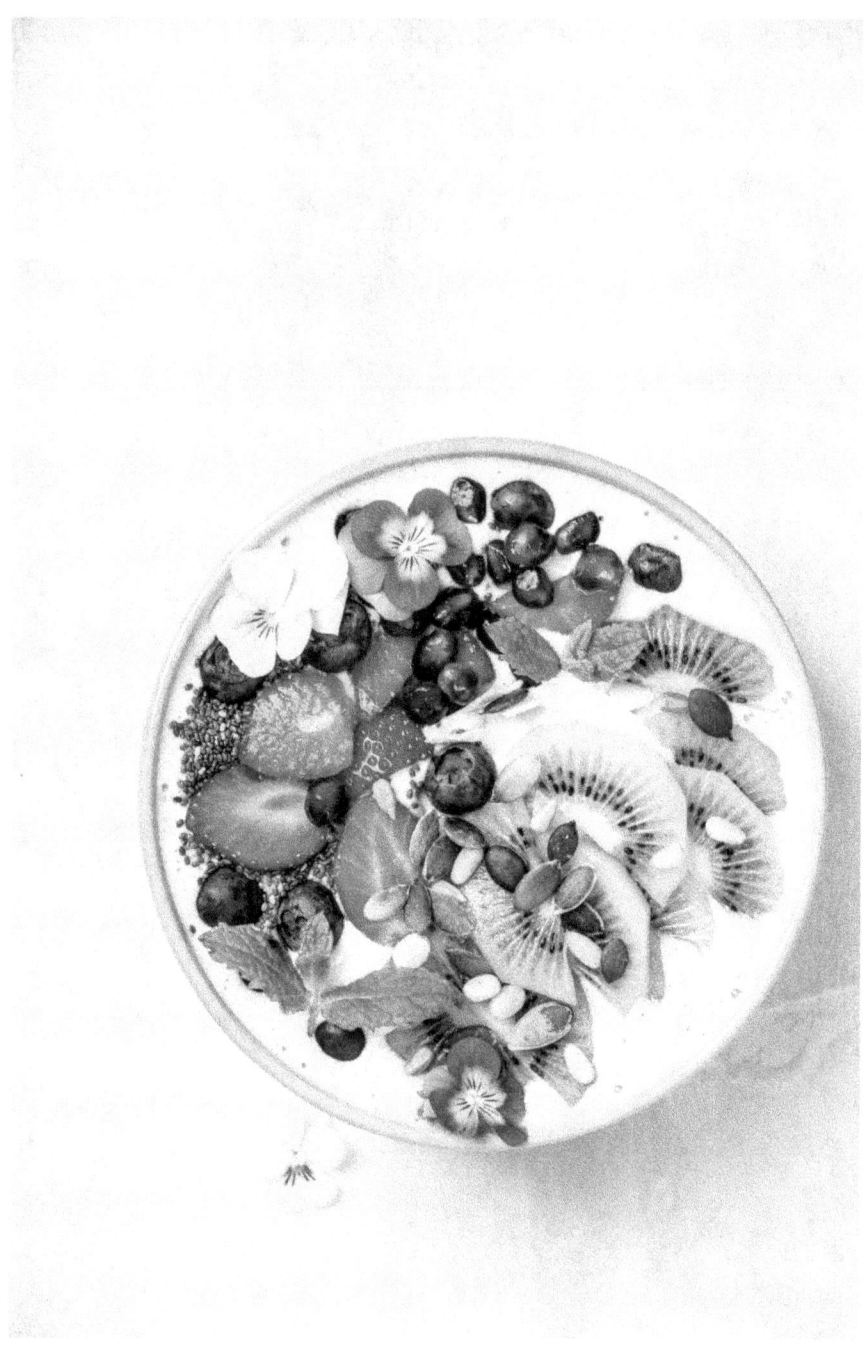

INTRODUCTION

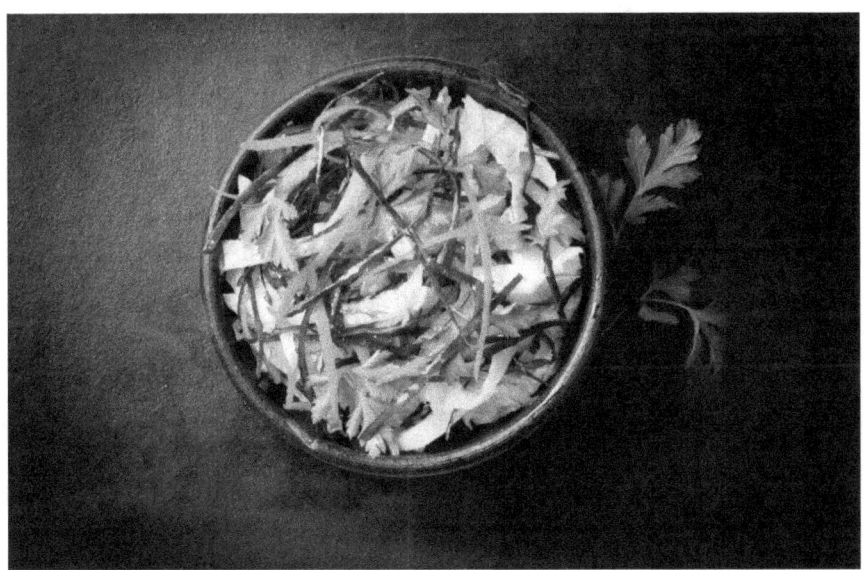

What does it mean to be a vegetarian?

A Vegetarian is a person who does not eat meat, poultry, or fish. Vegetarians eat only plant foods such as fruits, vegetables, legumes, and grains or products made from them. Some people think of a vegetarian as a person who does not eat red meat but may consume fish and chicken. Other people consider a vegetarian to be someone who avoids eating all animal flesh, including fish, poultry, and red meat. However, "true" vegetarians avoid the consumption of all meats, including fish and chicken.

Vegetarianism is not a new concept; it has been practiced since ancient times in India during the Vedic period (1500-500 BC) as well as in Greece and Rome. It continues to be practiced today in modern society around the world. In most cases, it is a matter of individual choice.

Eating meat and fish has been a common practice all over the world for thousands of years. In some cultures, the preparation of the meat or fish symbolizes wealth and luxury, while in others it represents a source of survival. Today, people are becoming more aware of the impact that their food choices have on their health as well as on the environment.

Why do people become vegetarians? The reasons vary widely from person to person. Some people object to the cruelty and suffering of animals raised for food. Some people object to the environmental effects of producing meat and fish. Others become vegetarians because they believe animal flesh is unhealthy to eat or because they believe it is unspiritual or unwise. For some, it is a choice of economic necessity.

How often should you eat fruits and vegetables? The recommendation is to eat five servings per day based on a 2,000 calorie diet. One serving is equal to one-half cup raw or one cup ready-to-eat. Fruits and vegetables provide vitamins, minerals, fiber, and other nutrients that are essential for good health. It is recommended that most Americans make fruits and vegetables the basis of their diet; ideally, they should be eaten at every meal.

So, specifically, what are the foods that one needs to avoid? These are as follows:

- Beef
- Pork
- Lamb
- Veal
- All Game (deer, elk, etc.)
- Any other land mammal that's been fed animal products or by-products such as eggs and dairy (many land mammals are herbivores)
- Fish and Shellfish
- Goose and Duck

- Emu and Alligator
- Any other animal that is not a seafood product
- Animal by-products such as gelatin (e.g., gummy bears)

As a vegetarian, what specific foods do you avoid? For starters, you can limit your consumption of the following:

- Pork and bacon
- Eggs (or eat only eggs that are certified organic or non-cage free)
- Dairy products (or consume only dairy products that are certified organic)
- All products that are made from animals, such as leather shoes, belts, jackets, etc.

What are the substitutes that you use to replace the meat and fish that you avoid?

- Tofu (made from soybeans)
- Tempeh (made from soybeans)
- TVP (textured vegetable protein)
- Seitan (very high in protein, available as steak strips or chicken-style pieces)
- Soy Nuggets/Sausage

Being a vegetarian has its benefits, but there are definitely some challenges as well. If you are considering the option of being a vegetarian, the most important thing to consider is your overall health. However, if you have concerns with the lack of protein in your diet, believe that it's unwise to eat only plant products, or simply crave meat and fish and think you can't give them up without feeling hungry or deprived, then the choice of becoming a vegetarian may not be the right one for you.

This vegetarian cookbook will help you get a delicious and healthy recipe on the table that will make your life less stressful. A good recipe doesn't need a long list of ingredients to make it tasty, and while preparing meals may seem hard. You can eat together a healthy family food in the same amount of time you'd need to order takeout!

This vegetarian cookbook will show you a variety of dishes you can make with easy-to-find ingredients. This is the perfect practical guide for anyone looking to make a variety of delicious meals that are healthy. It includes recipes for breakfast, lunch, dinner, appetizers, and desserts, as well as those for snacks and sides. Whether looking to lose weight or just eat more healthily, this cookbook will make it easier than ever before!

So, let us begin the journey.

CHAPTER 1:

BREAKFAST RECIPES

1. Stewed Collard Greens

Preparation Time: 10 minutes

Cooking Time: 20 minutes

Servings: 4

Ingredients:

- 1 tablespoon vegetable oil
- 1 yellow onion, diced
- 1 collard greens bunch, roughly chopped
- 2 cups vegetable broth
- 1 teaspoon smoked paprika
- 1 tablespoon cider vinegar

- ½ teaspoon hot sauce

- ⅛ teaspoon kosher salt

- ⅛ teaspoon freshly ground black pepper

Directions:

1. With the pressure cooker on the sauté or brown setting, heat the vegetable oil until it shimmers. Stir the onion and stir it frequently until it is softened and translucent, about 5 minutes. Add the collard greens, vegetable broth, and paprika.

2. Lock lid and set the timer for 20 minutes at high pressure. When the timer is off, naturally release it for 10 minutes. Then totally remove the lid after.

3. Stir in the vinegar, hot sauce, salt, and pepper. Serve hot.

4. To prepare the collard greens, rinse the leaves well by immersing them in a sink full of cool water. Fold leaves in half along the stem and use a chef's knife to cut away the toughest part of the stem. Then stack a few leaves at a time, roll them up into a cigar shape, and slice them into wide ribbons. You can further chop the ribbons if desired.

Nutrition: Calories: 30 Carbs: 6g Fat: 0g Protein: 2g

2. **Green Beans, Four Ways**

Preparation Time: 10 minutes

Cooking Time: 2 minutes

Servings: 4

Ingredients:

- 1 cup water
- 4 pounds green beans, trimmed
- Salt and pepper
- 2 teaspoons extra-virgin olive oil
- 2 tablespoons finely grated parmesan cheese
- 1 cup mixed sliced mushrooms
- ¼ cup packaged fried onions
- ¼ cup toasted slivered almonds
- 2 teaspoons sesame oil over
- 1 tablespoon toasted sesame seeds

Directions:

1. Add the water to the pressure cooker pot. Place a steamer insert in the cooker. Place the beans in the steamer insert.

2. Lock lid and set the timer for 2 minutes at high pressure. When the timer is off, quick release the pressure and open the lid. Use tongs to transfer the beans to a serving bowl.

3. Season the beans with one of the following:

4. Toss beans with salt, pepper, 2 teaspoons extra-virgin olive oil, and 2 tablespoons finely grated Parmesan cheese.

5. Place 1 tablespoon of unsalted butter on the hot beans and add salt and pepper. Toss with tongs to melt the butter and coat the beans. Sprinkle with ¼ cup toasted slivered almonds.

6. Drizzle 2 teaspoons of sesame oil over the beans and add salt and pepper. Toss the beans with tongs to coat them with the oil. Sprinkle the toasted 1 tablespoon sesame seeds on the top of the beans.

7. Sauté 1 cup mixed sliced mushrooms in butter until softened, 6 to 7 minutes. Stir the mushrooms into the beans and add salt and pepper. Top with ¼ cup packaged fried onions.

8. To prepare green beans, break or trim the ends off each bean. You can do this by lining up a handful of beans on the cutting board and using a sharp knife to cut off all the ends at once.

Nutrition: Calories: 40 Carbs: 9g Fat: 0g Protein: 2g

3. **Maple-Glazed Carrots**

Preparation Time: 8 minutes

Cooking Time: 2 minutes

Servings: 4

Ingredients:

- 1 cup water
- 1 pound baby carrots
- 1½ tablespoons unsalted butter
- 1½ tablespoons pure maple syrup
- ¼ teaspoon kosher salt
- Pinch freshly ground black pepper
- 1 teaspoon fresh minced thyme

Directions:

1. Place the water and carrots in the pot of a pressure cooker.
2. Then lock the lid and set the timer for 2 minutes at high pressure. When the timer is done, release quickly the pressure, open the cooker and switch to the brown setting.

3. Put the butter, maple syrup, salt, and pepper, then sauté the carrots for 2 to 3 minutes or until the remaining liquid almost evaporates. Sprinkle with fresh thyme. Serve hot or warm.

Nutrition: Calories: 110 Carbs: 0g Fat: 4g Protein: 1g

4. **Beets, Two Ways**

Preparation Time: 10 minutes

Cooking Time: 12 to 16 minutes

Servings: 4

Ingredients:

- 1 cup of water
- 1 pound medium-size beets, root, and stems trimmed

For Version 1

- 2 tablespoons unsalted butter
- 2 tablespoons granulated sugar
- 2 tablespoons apple cider vinegar
- ⅛ teaspoon kosher salt
- Pinch freshly ground black pepper

For Version 2

- 2 tablespoons unsalted butter
- ⅛ teaspoon kosher salt

- Pinch freshly ground black pepper
- ¼ cup finely grated Parmesan cheese
- 1 tablespoon minced fresh parsley

Directions:

1. Place a steamer insert or a rack in the pot of a pressure cooker. Add the water to the cooker. Place the beets on the steamer insert.

2. Lock on the lid and then set the timer for 13 minutes at high pressure, less if the beets are very small. When the timer is done, release the pressure and open the lid. Check the beets using a fork; the fork should easily pierce the beets, which should still be firm but a bit of softness when squeezed. If they still seem very hard, like an uncooked potato, lock the lid back on and cook at high pressure for 3 more minutes.

3. When the beets are ready and cooked, remove them from the cooker with tongs and let them rest until cool enough. Slip off the skins from the beets, they should come right off. Quarter the beets and slice into bite-size pieces.

4. To prepare version 1, remove the rack and pour the water out of the pressure cooker. With the setting on sauté or brown, melt the butter. Add the sugar and vinegar and then stir until the sugar dissolves. Add the beets and stir to coat them evenly with the vinegar mixture. Add the salt and pepper. Serve hot or warm. (Note: If you want to serve this recipe chilled, replace the butter with extra-virgin olive oil; otherwise, the butter will congeal.)

5. To prepare version 2, place the hot sliced beets into a bowl and toss with the butter, salt, and pepper. When the butter is already melted, and it coats the beets, add now the Parmesan and parsley and toss to distribute.

Nutrition: Calories: 154 Carbs: 20g Fat: 6g Protein: 5g

5. Crustless Spinach Quiche

Preparation Time: 10 minutes

Cooking Time: 5 hours

Servings: 6

Ingredients:

- Nonstick cooking spray
- 4 large eggs
- 1 cup half-and-half
- 1 cup shredded sharp Cheddar cheese
- 3 cups fresh baby spinach leaves
- 2 cups cubed ham
- ½ teaspoon salt
- ¼ teaspoon freshly ground black pepper

Directions:

1. Prepare a nonstick slow cooker and spray it with cooking spray.

2. In a large bowl, beat the eggs. Add the half-and-half, Cheddar cheese, spinach, ham, salt, and pepper, and stir to combine. Pour the mixture into your slow cooker.

3. Cover your slow cooker. Cook for 5 hours on low or 3 hours on high.

4. Turn off the slow cooker and let it sit for 15 minutes before serving.

5. Empty a box of frozen spinach into a colander. Run warm water over the spinach until it's warm. Use a clean a paper towel or a towel to press down on the spinach and release as much water as possible.

Nutrition: Calories: 381 Total Fat: 27g Fat: 14g Cholesterol: 277mg Carbohydrates: 7g Fiber: 1g Protein: 27g

6. Blueberry-Coconut Quinoa

Preparation Time: 10 minutes

Cooking Time: 3 hours

Servings: 4

Ingredients:

- ¾ cup quinoa, rinsed and drained
- ¼ cup shredded unsweetened coconut
- 1 tablespoon honey
- 1 (13.5-ounce) can coconut milk
- 2 cups fresh blueberries

Directions:

1. Put the rinsed quinoa in the slow cooker. Sprinkle the coconut over the top and then drizzle with the honey.

2. Open the can of coconut milk. Stir until smooth and even in consistency. Pour over the quinoa.

3. Cover your slow cooker and cook for 3 hours on low.

4. Stir the quinoa, then scoop it into four serving bowls. Top each bowl with blueberries and serve.

5. If fresh blueberries are out of season or aren't available, you can easily substitute frozen blueberries, which are available year-round.

Nutrition: Calories: 468 Total Fat: 33g Carbohydrates: 43g Fiber: 7g Protein: 8g

7. Apple-Cinnamon Oatmeal

Preparation Time: 10 minutes

Cooking Time: 4 hours

Servings: 4

Ingredients:

- 1 cup steel-cut oats
- 1 tablespoon unsalted butter, melted
- 4 cups water
- ¼ cup brown sugar
- 1 teaspoon ground cinnamon
- ½ teaspoon salt
- 1 Granny Smith apple, peeled, cored, and chopped
- ½ cup milk

Directions:

1. Combine the steel-cut oats and butter in the slow cooker. Stir the oats until it is coated with the butter. Add the water, brown sugar, cinnamon, and salt.

2. Cover your slow cooker for it to cook for 4 hours at low.

3. Stir the chopped apple into the oatmeal. Scoop into four serving bowls and serve with a splash of milk.

Nutrition: Calories: 143 Total Fat: 4g Cholesterol: 10mg Sodium: 329mg Carbohydrates: 25g Fiber: 3g Protein: 3g

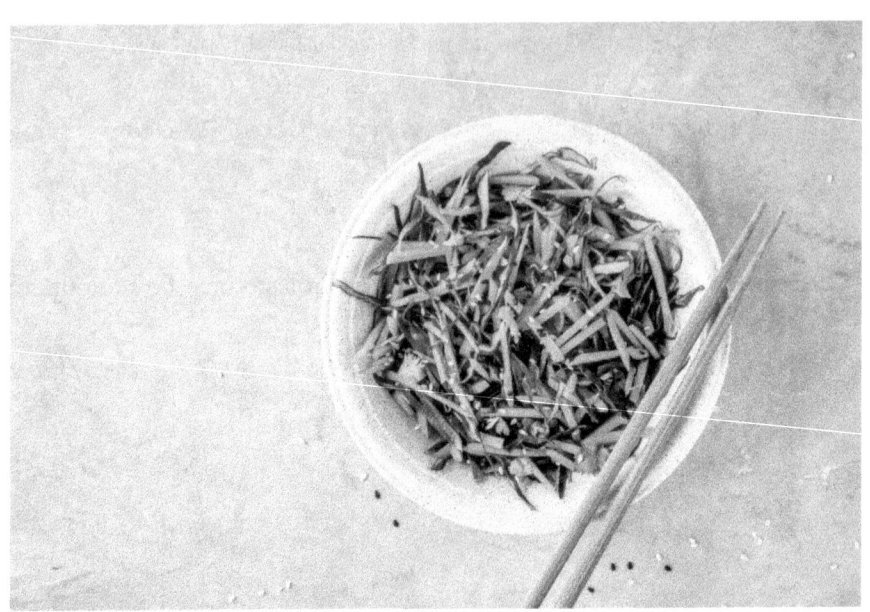

CHAPTER 2:

LUNCH RECIPES

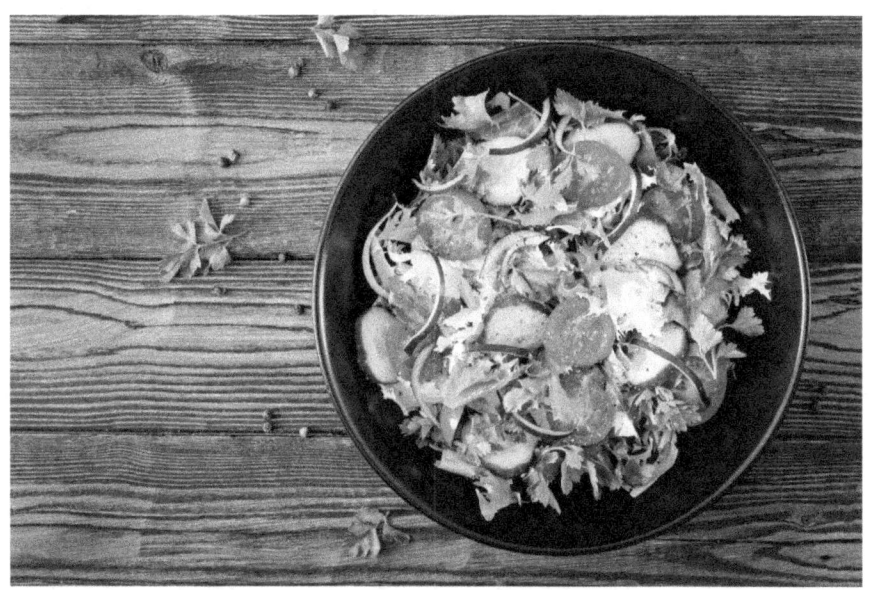

8. Mexican Beans

Preparation Time: 15 minutes

Cooking Time: 35 minutes

Servings: 2

Ingredients:

- ½ cup dried pinto beans
- 2 cups water
- 1 small onion, chopped
- 1 medium ripe tomato, chopped
- 1 fresh bell pepper, chopped
- 1 tablespoon fresh cilantro, chopped

Directions:

1. Select the High Sauté setting on the Instant Pot, add pinto beans, water, onion, ripe tomato, and bell pepper. Secure the lid. Press the Cancel button to reset the program, then select the Pressure Cook or Manual setting and set the cooking time for 35 minutes at High Pressure.

2. Let the pressure release naturally; this will take 10 to 20 minutes.

3. Garnish with fresh cilantro.

Nutrition: Calories 212 Fat 0.9g Cholesterol 0mg Carbohydrate 40.4g Fiber 9.8g

9. Lime-Mint Soup

Preparation Time: 5 minutes

Cooking Time: 30 minutes

Servings: 4

Ingredients:

- 4 cups vegetable broth
- ¼ cup fresh mint leaves,
- ¼ cup chopped scallions
- 3 garlic cloves
- 3 tablespoons freshly squeezed lime juice

Directions:

1. In a large stockpot, combine the broth, mint, scallions, garlic, and lime juice. Bring to a boil over medium-high heat.
2. Cover the pot and reduce the heat to low. Let it simmer for 15 minutes and serve.

Nutrition: Calories: 55 Fat: 2g Carbohydrates: 5g Fiber: 1g Protein: 5g

10. Lemony Kale Salad

Preparation Time: 10 minutes Cooking Time: 30 minutes

Servings: 4

Ingredients:

- 2 tablespoons freshly squeezed lemon juice
- ½ tablespoon maple syrup
- 1 teaspoon minced garlic
- 5 cups chopped kale

Directions:

1. Add the lemon juice, maple syrup, and garlic together in a large bowl. Add the kale, massage it in the dressing for 1 to 2 minutes, and serve.

2. Preparation Tip: Make sure to thoroughly massage the kale with the dressing ingredients. This will give the kale a beautiful texture and get the lemon and garlic flavors properly incorporated.

Nutrition: Calories: 51 Fat: 0g Carbohydrates: 11g Fiber: 1g

CHAPTER 3:

MAIN MEALS RECIPES

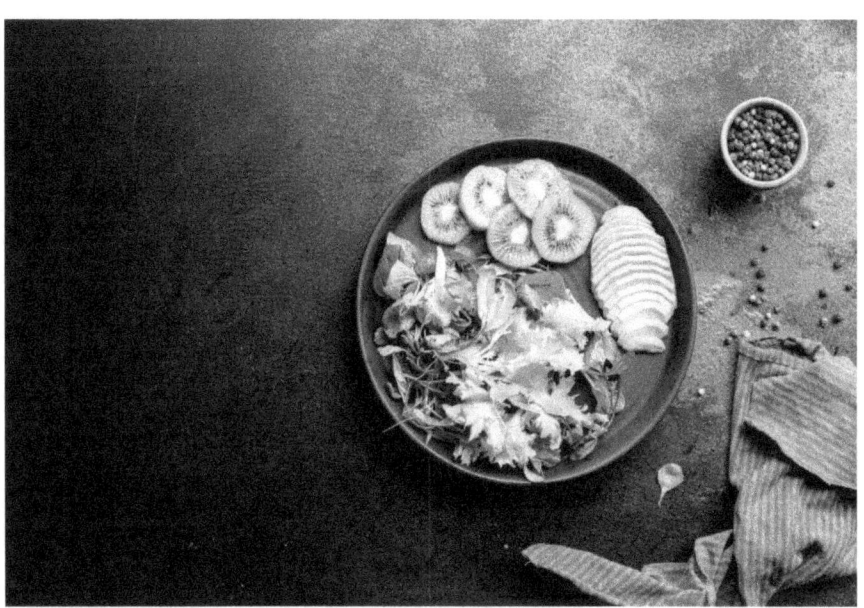

11. Moroccan Chickpea Rolls

Preparation Time: 10 minutes

Cooking Time: 25 minutes

Servings: 6

Ingredients:

- 5 cups Chickpeas (cooked or canned)
- ¼ cup full-flat coconut milk
- ¼ copra's El Han out

Directions:

1. Now with the chickpeas, soak, then cook 1½ cup of dry chickpeas according to the procedure if necessary.
2. Prepare oven, then preheat it to 350°F/175°C, then line a baking sheet using the parchment paper.
3. Add chickpeas and other spices to the food processor. Slowly pour in the coconut milk to form a chunky mixture.
4. Mash chickpeas and spices in a large bowl and then add the coconut milk and knead everything into a chunky mixture.

5. Get a handful of chickpea mixture, then knead into a log shape, make sure it is 4 inches long and also 2 inches thick.

6. Make until you have 16 rolls in totality.

7. Place the rolled chickpeas on the baking sheet, and bake for 15 minutes.

8. Get the baking sheet off the oven and turn the rolls over, then bake for another 10 minutes.

9. Take the rolls out of the oven once cooked. Make sure it is brown and crispy. Let it cool down.

10. Serve the rolls with the optional toppings.

Nutrition: Calories: 490 Carbs: 75.3 g. Fat: 10.3 g. Protein: 24 g.

12. Smoky Cajun Bowl

Preparation Time: 10 minutes

Cooking Time: 25 minutes

Servings: 4

Ingredients:

- 2 cups Black beans (cooked or canned)
- 1 cup Quick-cooking brown rice (dry)
- 1 7-ounces pack Smoked tofu (cubed)
- 2 cups Tomato cubes (canned or fresh)
- 1 tablespoon Salt-free Cajun spices

Directions:

1. When using dry beans, make sure to soak and cook ⅔ cup (113 g.) of dry black beans according to the procedure. Cook brown rice base and using package instructions.

2. Put the pan over medium-high heat. Add tofu cubes, tomato cubes, and you can also add ¼ cup of water.

3. Stir until everything is cooked. Afterward, add the black beans, cooked brown rice, and Cajun spices.

4. Turn heat off, then stir occasionally for 5 minutes until heated through.

5. Then divide the smoky Cajun beans and rice between 4 bowls, serve with the optional toppings, and enjoy

6. Store smoky Cajun beans and rice in an airtight container in the fridge, and you can consume it within 3 days. You can also store for a maximum of 30 days in the fridge and thaw at room temperature. You can use a microwave, toaster oven, or non-stick frying pan to reheat the smoky Cajun beans and rice.

Nutrition: Calories: 371 Carbs: 60.6 g Fat: 5 g. Protein: 19.6 g.

13. Sloppy Cajun Burgers

Preparation Time: 10 minutes

Cooking Time: 5 minutes

Servings: 4

Ingredients:

- 1 cup Black beans (cooked or canned)
- 1 7-ounces pack textured soy mince
- 1 cup Tomato cubes (canned or fresh)
- ¼ cup Salt-free Cajun spices
- 4 whole wheat buns

Directions:

1. When using dry beans, make sure to soak and cook ⅓ cup (56 g.) of dry black beans according to the method
2. Put the non-stick deep frying pan on medium-high heat and add the soy mince and the tomato cubes.
3. Cook for about 3 minutes and stir occasionally until everything is cooked.

4. Add the black beans and Cajun spices and let it cook for another 2 minutes while stirring.

5. Turn off the heat and divide the bottom halves of the buns between 2 plates.

6. Transfer a quarter of the sloppy Cajun mix onto each of the bun halves and add the optional toppings.

7. Cover each burger with the other bun half, serve right away and enjoy!

8. Store the sloppy Cajun mix in an airtight container in the fridge and consume within 2 days. You can store in the freezer for a maximum of 60 days and thaw at room temperature. The sloppy Cajun mix can be served cold or reheated in a microwave or a saucepan.

Nutrition: Calories: 134 Carbs: 15.8 g. Fat: 0.7 g. Protein: 14.7 g.

CHAPTER 4:

VEGETABLES, SALADS AND SIDES RECIPES

14. Garlic Roasted Carrots

Preparation Time: 5 minutes

Cooking Time: 40 minutes

Servings: 6

Ingredients:

- 24 baby carrots (tops 2-inches trimmed)
- 2 tablespoons balsamic vinegar
- 5 cloves minced garlic
- 1 tablespoon thyme (dried)

- 2 tablespoons parsley leaves (chopped)

What you'll need from store cupboard

- 2 tablespoons olive oil
- Kosher salt to taste
- Black pepper (freshly ground) to taste

Directions:

1. Preheat your oven to 350 F.
2. Coat a baking sheet with nonstick spray.
3. Place carrots on the baking sheet in a single layer.
4. Add vinegar, olive oil, garlic, and thyme, then season with pepper and salt.
5. Toss gently to combine, then place in the oven.
6. Bake for about 40 minutes until tender.
7. Garnish with parsley and serve immediately. Enjoy!

Nutrition: Calories: 59.5 Fat: 4.6g Carbs: 4.3g Protein: 0.4g

15. Baked Parmesan Mushrooms

Preparation Time: 10 minutes

Cooking Time: 15 minutes

Servings: 4

Ingredients:

- 1½ pound cremini mushrooms, thinly sliced
- ¼ cup lemon juice (freshly squeezed)
- 3 minced garlic cloves
- ¼ cup parmesan (grated)
- 2 tablespoons thyme (dried)

What you'll need from store cupboard

- 3 tablespoons olive oil
- Kosher salt to taste
- Black pepper (freshly ground) to taste

Directions:

1. Preheat your oven to 350 F.

2. Coat a baking sheet with nonstick spray.

3. Place mushrooms on the baking sheet in a single layer.

4. Add olive oil, lemon zest, lemon juice, garlic, parmesan, and thyme, then season with pepper and salt.

5. Combine and place in the oven.

6. Set baking for 15 minutes or until tender and brown. Toss occasionally.

7. Serve immediately and enjoy.

Nutrition: Calories: 163.5 Fat: 12.2g Carbs: 10.3g Protein: 6.9g

16. Buttery Garlic Green Beans

Preparation Time: 10 minutes

Cooking Time: 10 minutes

Servings: 4

Ingredients:

- 1 pound trimmed and halved fresh green beans
- 3 minced garlic cloves
- 2 pinches lemon pepper

What you'll need from store cupboard

- 3 tablespoons butter
- Salt to taste

Directions:

1. Place fresh green beans in a skillet (large) then cover with water. Boil over medium-high heat.
2. Reduce to medium-low heat and simmer the beans for about 5 minutes until beans soften lightly.

3. Drain excess water, then add butter and cook for about 3 minutes while stirring until butter melts.

4. Add garlic, stir and cook for about 4 minutes until garlic is fragrant and tender.

5. Season with salt and lemon pepper.

Nutrition: Calories: 116 Fat: 8.8g Carbs: 8.9g Protein: 2.3g

17. Roasted Butternut Squash Puree

Preparation Time: 15 minutes

Cooking Time: 45 minutes

Servings: 4

Ingredients:

- 1 large seeded and halved butternut squash
- 2 cups chicken stock

What you'll need from store cupboard

- Salt to taste
- Black pepper (ground) to taste

Directions:

1. Preheat your oven to 400 F.
2. Place squash on a baking sheet.
3. Roast squash for 45-60 minutes in the oven until slightly brown and tender. Cool until it can be easily handled.
4. Put squash into a blender and blend until smooth.
5. Add ¼ cup chicken stock at a time while blending until smooth.

6. Season with pepper and salt. Serve and enjoy.

Nutrition: Calories: 159 Fat: 0.6g Carbs: 40.3g Protein: 3.7g

18. Irish Bombay Potatoes

Preparation Time: 5 minutes

Cooking Time: 30 minutes

Servings: 4

Ingredients:

- 35 ounces potato, peeled
- 2 tablespoons curry paste
- 2 tablespoons tomato paste
- ½ cup basil, fresh
- 1 garlic clove

What you'll need from the store cupboard

- 1 tbsp salt
- 4 tablespoons oil
- 2 tablespoons curry powder
- 2 tablespoons white vinegar

Directions:

1. Heat your oven to 390F.

2. Quarter the peeled potatoes then place them in a mixing bowl.

3. Add curry paste, tomato paste, salt, oil, curry powder, then mix until the potatoes ate well coated.

4. Layer the potatoes on your oven tray and bake them for fifteen minutes.

5. Add fresh basil and garlic five minutes before the end of cooking. Mix well.

6. Serve with dips. Enjoy.

Nutrition: Calories 288 Fat 14g Carbs 33g, Protein 7g

19. Healthy Mashed Sweet Potato

Preparation Time: 5 minutes

Cooking Time: 20 minutes

Servings: 2

Ingredients:

- 2 sweet potatoes, peeled and chopped
- 2 garlic cloves
- 1 thumb ginger, fresh
- 1 chili pepper
- 1 handful coriander, fresh

What you'll need from the store cupboard

- 6 tablespoons olive oil
- ½ juiced lime

Directions:

1. Add sweet potatoes to boiling and salted water in a saucepan. Let the sweet potatoes cook for twenty minutes.

2. Meanwhile, add olive oil to a small pan. Add chopped garlic cloves and ginger.

3. Make an incision on the chili pepper, or make four incisions on the chili pepper if you like your food spicier.

4. Let the three fry in oil for some few minutes.

5. When the sweet potatoes are cooked, poke them with a knife to make sure they are fully soft.

6. Add the potatoes to the pan and use a spoon to remove the garlic, ginger, and chili pieces from the oil. The heat should be off.

7. Mash all them together until smooth.

8. Serve with coriander and lime juice. Enjoy.

Nutrition: Calories 503 Fat 42g Carbs 31g Protein 2g

20. Spinach Tomato Quesadilla

Preparation Time: 5 minutes

Cooking Time: 10 minutes

Servings: 2

Ingredients:

- 2 whole-grain tortillas
- ½ cup cheddar cheese, sliced
- 1 cup mozzarella cheese, sliced
- 1 tomato
- 1 ½ cup spinach

What you'll need from the store cupboard

- 1 tablespoon homemade pesto

Directions:

1. Spread a layer of homemade pesto over half tortilla.
2. Add a cheese layer on the tortilla.
3. Slice the tomato and a layer on the cheese.

4. Add a layer of spinach on top, then finally another cheese layer

5. Put half of the tortilla on top.

6. Place the tortilla on a hot pan, cover the pan, and heat for four minutes on each side. The cheese should have melted. Serve and enjoy.

Nutrition: Calories 386 Fat 19g Carbs 26g Protein 23g

21. Lentil Tacos

Preparation Time: 5minutes

Cooking Time: minutes

Servings: 6

Ingredients:

- 1 onion, diced
- 2 garlic cloves, diced
- 1 cup brown lentils, cooked
- 2 tablespoons burrito seasoning
- 2 taco shells

What you'll need from the store cupboard

- 2 tablespoons olive oil
- 4 cups of water
- 6 tablespoons salsa
- 1 ½ cups mixed salad
- ½ cup cherry tomatoes, sliced

Directions:

1. Heat olive oil in the saucepan, then fry the onions until soft.

2. Add diced garlic, then drain the lentils and add them.

3. Add seasoning and water, then stir well. Cook until all water has evaporated.

4. Put the taco shells for three minutes.

5. Layer the lentils at the bottom, followed by cheese if you desire, salsa, mixed salad, and finally, the cherry tomatoes. Serve and enjoy.

Nutrition: Calories 239 Fat 13g Carbs 20g Protein 9g

CHAPTER 5:

DESSERT RECIPES

22. Cardamom Date Bites

Preparation Time: 15 minutes, plus time to soak

Cooking Time: 15 minutes

Servings: 8

Ingredients:

- 1 cup pitted dates
- 3 cups old-fashioned rolled oats
- ¼ cup ground flaxseed
- 1 teaspoon ground cardamom
- 3 ripe bananas, mashed (about 1½ cups)

Directions:

1. Preheat the oven to 350°F. Line a baking sheet with parchment paper.

2. In a small bowl, place the dates and cover with hot water. Let it sit until softened, 10 to 30 minutes, depending on the dates, and then drain. Purée in a food processor or blender. Set the date paste aside.

3. In the food processor, grind the oats and ground flaxseed until they resemble flour.

4. In a large bowl, mix together the cardamom and mashed bananas. Stir in the ground oat-flaxseed mixture.

5. Form into walnut-size balls and flatten a little. Place on the baking sheet and form an indentation in the middle using a ¼ teaspoon measuring spoon. Fill each indentation with about ½ teaspoon of date paste.

6. Bake 15 minutes or until the bites are golden.

Nutrition: Calories: 82 Fat: 2g Carbohydrate: 16g Protein: 2g

23. Sweet Potato Pie Nice Cream

Preparation Time: 5 minutes

Cooking Time: 0 minutes

Servings: 2

Ingredients:

- 2 medium sweet potatoes, cooked (see here)
- ½ cup plant-based milk (here or here)
- 1 tablespoon maple syrup
- 1 teaspoon vanilla extract
- ½ teaspoon ground cinnamon

Directions:

1. Line a baking sheet with parchment paper.
2. Remove the skin from the cooked sweet potatoes and cut the flesh into 1-inch cubes. Place on the baking sheet in an even layer, then place in the freezer overnight, or for a minimum of 4 hours.

3. In a food processor, combine the frozen sweet potato, milk, maple syrup, vanilla, and cinnamon.

4. Process on medium speed for 1 to 2 minutes, or until the mixture has been blended into a smooth soft-serve consistency, and serve.

Nutrition: Calories: 155 Total fat: 1g Carbohydrates: 34g Fiber: 5g Protein: 2g

24. Peanut Butter Nice Cream

Preparation Time: 30 minutes

Cooking Time: 0 minutes

Servings: 2

Ingredients:

- 3 frozen ripe bananas, broken into thirds
- 3 tablespoons plant-based milk (here or here)
- 2 tablespoons defatted peanut powder
- 1 teaspoon vanilla extract

Directions:

1. Combine the bananas, milk, peanut powder, and vanilla in a food processor.
2. Process on medium speed for 30 to 60 seconds, or until the bananas have been blended into a smooth soft-serve consistency, and serve.

Nutrition: Calories: 237 Total fat: 3g Carbohydrates: 45g Fiber: 7g Protein: 10g

25. No Bake Apple Pie

Preparation Time: 5 minutes

Cooking Time: 0 minutes

Servings: 2

Ingredients:

- 2 chopped red apples
- ¼ cup chopped almonds
- ¼ cup sultanas
- 2 tsp. lemon juice
- ½ tsp. cinnamon

Directions:

1. In a bowl, mix the almonds, sultanas, lemon juice, and cinnamon. Toss the apples in the mixture, making sure the apples are completely covered.
2. Plate the dessert, top with a dollop of chilled coconut cream, garnish with some chopped almonds and serve.

Nutrition: Calories: 300 Total fat: 13g Carbohydrates: 17g Protein: 2g

26. Cashew-Chocolate Truffles

Preparation Time: 15 minutes

Cooking Time: 0 minutes

Servings: 12 truffles

Ingredients:

- 1 cup raw cashews, soaked in water overnight
- ¾ cup pitted dates
- 2 tablespoons coconut oil
- 1 cup unsweetened shredded coconut, divided
- 1 to 2 tablespoons cocoa powder, to taste

Directions:

1. In a food processor, combine the cashews, dates, coconut oil, ½ cup of shredded coconut, and cocoa powder. Pulse until fully incorporated; it will resemble chunky cookie dough.
2. Spread the remaining ½ cup of shredded coconut on a plate.
3. Form the mixture into tablespoon-size balls and roll on the plate to cover with the shredded coconut. Transfer to a parchment

paper-lined plate or baking sheet. Repeat to make 12 truffles. Place the truffles in the refrigerator for 1 hour to set.

4. Transfer the truffles to a storage container or freezer-safe bag and seal.

Nutrition: Calories: 238 Total fat: 18g Carbohydrates: 16g Protein: 3g

27. Crusty Rosemary Bread

Preparation Time: 10 minutes

Cooking Time: 3 hours and 50 minutes

Servings: 8

Ingredients:

- 10-ounce of all-purpose flour, leveled
- 1 teaspoon of nutritional yeast
- 1 1/2 teaspoons of salt
- 2 tablespoons of chopped rosemary, and more for sprinkling
- 2 tablespoons of olive oil, and more for brushing
- 1 cup of water, lukewarm

Directions:

1. Using a large bowl, place the flour and add the remaining ingredients except for water.
2. Stir properly, add 3/4 cup of water and stir again until the moist dough comes together. Add more water if need be.

3. Cover the bowl with a damp towel and let it sit for 30 minutes in a warm place.

4. Then knead the dough for 3 minutes, return it to the bowl, cover it with a damp cloth and let it sit for another 30 minutes in a warm place.

5. Massage the dough again for 3 minutes, return it to the bowl, cover it with a damp cloth and let it sit for another 2 to 3 hours in a warm place or until the dough expands double in size.

6. Transfers the dough to a clean working space covered with flour and mold it into balls.

7. Then take a large parchment sheet, sprinkle it with flour, and place the dough on it.

8. Brush the top of the dough with olive oil, sprinkle it with rosemary leaves, and lower it into a 6-quarts slow cooker.

9. Cover the top and let the dough rest for 1 hour.

10. Then plug in the slow cooker and let it cook at the high heat setting for 2 hours or until an inserted wooden skewer into the loaf comes out clean, while checking the dough at 45 minutes intervals.

11. Transfer the loaf into a preheated broiler and broil it for 5 minutes or until the top are nicely browned and crusty.

12. Let the loaf cool off on the wire rack before slicing to serve.

Nutrition: Calories: 190 Carbohydrates: 19g Protein: 5g Fats: 11g

28. Chewy Olive Parmesan Bread

Preparation Time: 10 minutes

Cooking Time: 4 hours

Servings: 8

Ingredients:

- 3 cups of bread flour, leveled
- 3/4 cup of diced olives
- 1/2 tablespoon of minced garlic
- 1 teaspoon of nutritional yeast
- 1/4 cup of grated vegetarian Parmesan cheese
- 1 1/2 cups of water

Directions:

1. Using a large bowl, place the flour and add the remaining ingredients except for water.

2. Stir properly, add some water and stir again until the moist dough comes together.

3. Cover the bowl with a damp towel and let it sit for 1 1/2 hours in a warm place or until the dough expands double in size.

4. Then take a large parchment sheet, sprinkle it with flour, and place the dough on it.

5. Shape the dough along with the parchment sheet into round balls, cover it with a plastic wrap and let it sit for another 30 minutes.

6. Plug in the slow cooker and let cook at the high heat setting.

7. Drop the dough wrapped in the parchment sheet into the slow cooker and tuck to fit into it properly.

8. Cover the top with a wrapped dish towel or parchment sheets and let it cook for 2 hours at the high heat setting or until an inserted wooden skewer into the loaf comes out clean.

9. Transfer the loaf into a preheated oven at 400 degrees F and bake for 15 to 20 minutes or until the top is nicely browned and crusty.

10. Let the loaf cool off on a wire rack before slicing to serve.

Nutrition: Calories: 110 Carbohydrates: 14g Protein: 2g Fats: 6g

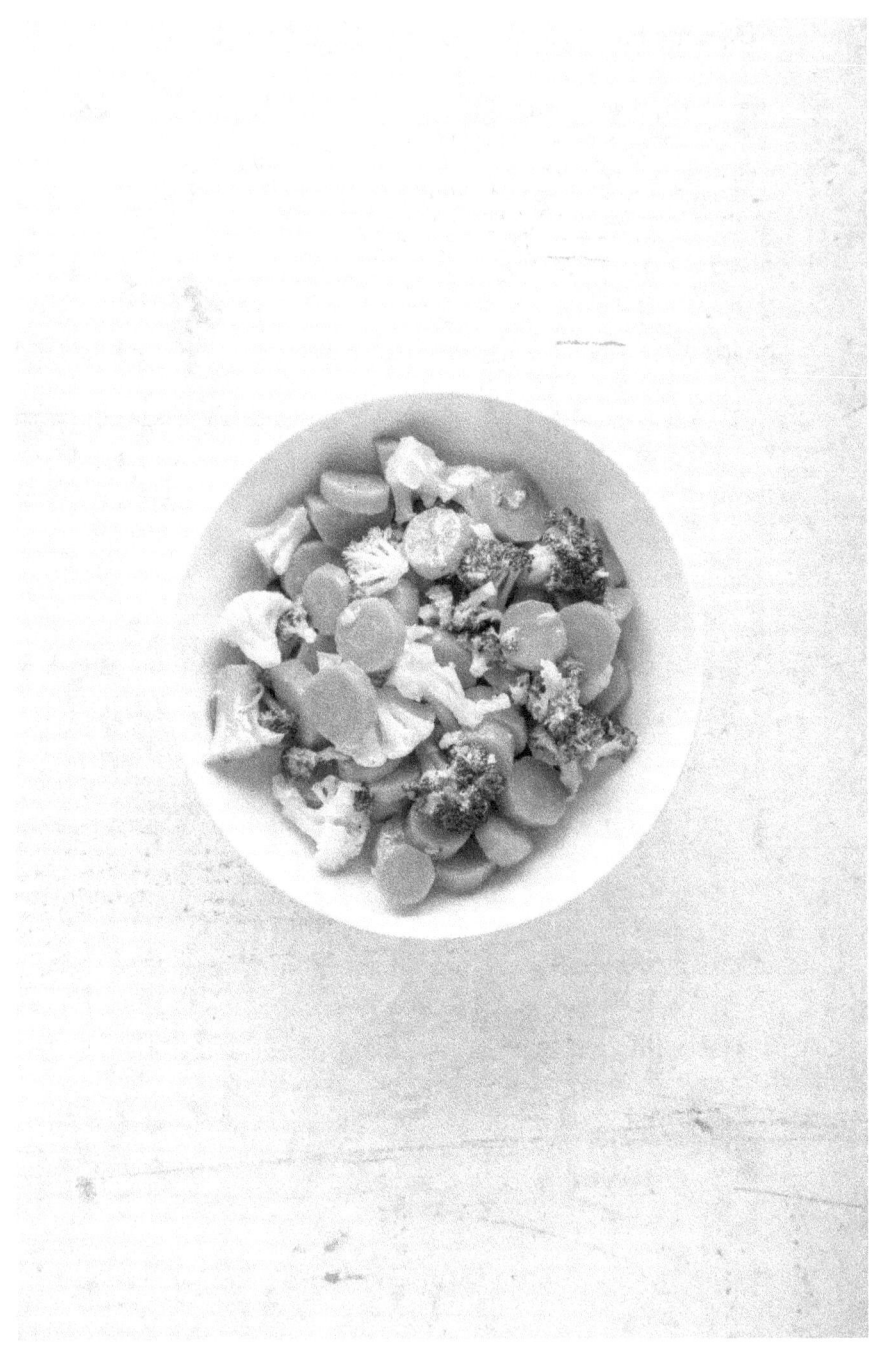

CHAPTER 6:

SNACK RECIPES

29. Baked Potatoes with Avocado Pico de Gallo

Preparation Time: 5 minutes

Cooking Time: 8 hours

Servings: 6

Ingredients:

- 6 russet potatoes

- ⅓ Cup red onion

- 1 ripe avocado, finely chopped

- ⅓ Cup fresh cilantro

- 4 Roma tomatoes, finely chopped

- 2 tablespoons olive oil

- Salt

- Black pepper

Directions:

1. Rinse the potatoes thoroughly, then dry with paper towels.

2. Poke the russet potatoes using a fork in several places. Rub it with olive oil. Wrap each potato tightly in aluminum foil. Put the potatoes in the slow cooker.

3. Cover the slow cooker, then cook for 8 hours on low, or until the potatoes are tender. Remove potatoes from the slow cooker. Cover the potatoes in a bowl using a clean towel to keep warm.

4. Now, prepare the pico de gallo. Gently mix and stir the onion, tomatoes, cilantro, and avocado in a bowl. Season with salt and pepper.

5. Unwrap each potato and halve lengthwise. Fluff the potato flesh with a fork. Top each potato with a generous portion of pico de gallo and serve.

Nutrition: Calories: 410 Total Fat: 12g Sodium: 50mg Carbohydrates: 72g Fiber: 8g Protein: 9g

30. Flourless Dark Chocolate Cake

Preparation Time: 10 minutes

Cooking Time: 45 minutes

Servings: 6

Ingredients:

- ½ cup of water
- ¾ cup coconut sugar or granulated sugar
- ⅛ Teaspoon of sea salt
- 1¼ pounds bittersweet chocolate (containing at least 60% cacao), roughly chopped
- 1 cup salted butter, cut into 1-inch cubes, plus more for greasing pan
- 7 eggs
- 2 teaspoons pure vanilla extract

Directions:

1. Preheat the oven to 300°F. Grease the springform pan for a 9-inch round and set the pan on a piece of foil. Fold the foil up outside of the pan, forming a waterproof layer. Set aside.

2. Combine the water, sugar, and salt over medium-high heat, stirring in a small saucepan, until the sugar is completely dissolved. Take off the pan from the heat and set it aside.

3. Place the chocolate in a large bowl over a medium saucepan of simmering water and stir until the chocolate has melted.

4. Get the chocolate from the heat. Beat in the butter one at a time using a hand mixer on medium speed until blended.

5. Beat in the sugar mixture and the eggs (one at a time) at medium speed. Add the vanilla and beat until smooth.

6. Prepared springform pan, then place the butter and place the pan into a larger pan. In a larger pan, bring the water to boil until it reaches one inch up the sides of the springform pan.

7. Bake until the edges are firm, about 45 minutes. Take the cake out of the oven and let cool on a rack.

8. Chill the cake in the refrigerator overnight. Remove from the springform pan when ready to serve.

9. Flavor Boost Chocolate and coffee are a popular pairing because the bitterness and sweetness create incredible richness. Stir one tablespoon of espresso powder into the water in step 2 along with the sugar and salt. Then follow the remaining steps as written.

Nutrition: Calories: 416 Fat: 30g Protein: 6g Cholesterol: 138mg Sodium: 192mg Carbohydrates: 40g Fiber: 3g

31. Creamy Peach Ice Pops

Preparation Time: 10 minutes

Cooking Time: 0 minutes

Servings: 8

Ingredients:

- 1 (14-ounce) can light coconut milk
- 2 peaches, peeled, pitted, and roughly chopped
- ¼ cup honey
- Pinch cinnamon

Directions:

1. In a blender, blend the coconut milk, peaches, honey, and cinnamon until smooth.
2. Pour the mixture into ice pop molds and freeze for about 5 hours.
3. Can stored for a week in the freezer using plastic wrap over the open tops of the molds.

4. Substitution Tip: You can create a staggering variety of wonderful flavors by swapping out the peaches for other ingredients—you'll need about 3 cups total. Try peeled plums, watermelon, cantaloupe, berries, sweet potato, mango, pineapple, and papaya in any combination or alone. Add an amount of honey, depending on the sweetness of the base ingredient.

Nutrition: Calories: 79 Total Fat: 3g Protein: 0g Cholesterol: 0mg Sodium: 4mg Carbohydrates: 13g Fiber: 1g

32. Melon-Lime Sorbet

Preparation Time: 15 minutes

Cooking Time: 0 minutes

Servings: 8

Ingredients:

- 1 small honeydew melon, cut into 1-inch chunks
- 1 small cantaloupe, cut into 1-inch chunks
- 2 tablespoons honey
- 2 tablespoons freshly squeezed lime juice
- Pinch cinnamon
- Water as needed

Directions:

1. Spread the honeydew and cantaloupe out on a baking sheet lined with parchment paper, then place in the freezer for up to 4 to 6 hours or until frozen.
2. In a food processor, add the frozen melon chunks and the honey, lime juice, and cinnamon.

3. Pulse and wait until smooth, add water (a tablespoon at a time) if needed to purée the melon.

4. Transfer the mixture to a container that is resalable and place in the freezer until set, about 30 minutes.

5. Substitution Tip: Almost any fruit will work in this recipe. You can try watermelon, peaches, plums, mangos, or berries. Some fruit has more water in it than others, so if you're using produce that's less juicy, add extra water or apple juice to create a smooth purée.

Nutrition: Calories: 97 Total Fat: 0g Protein: 2g Cholesterol: 0mg Sodium: 39mg Carbohydrates: 25g Fiber: 2g

33. Mandarin Ambrosia

Preparation Time: 5 minutes Cooking Time: 0 minutes

Servings: 6

Ingredients:

- ½ cup coconut cream, chilled in the refrigerator overnight
- 3 cups vegan mini marshmallows
- 1 cup shredded unsweetened coconut
- 3 small tangerines, peeled and segmented
- ½ cup sour cream

Directions:

1. In a large bowl, beat the cold coconut cream until it forms stiff peaks.
2. Stir in the marshmallows, coconut, tangerine segments, and sour cream until well mixed.
3. Place it in the refrigerator for 3 hours before serving.

Nutrition: Calories: 285 Total Fat: 22g Saturated Fat: 19g Protein: 4g Cholesterol: 6mg Sodium: 13mg Carbohydrates: 27g Fiber: 3g

34. Coconut-Quinoa Pudding

Preparation Time: 5 minutes

Cooking Time: 20 minutes

Servings: 6

Ingredients:

- 2 cups almond milk

- 1½ cups quinoa

- 1 cup light coconut milk

- ½ cup maple syrup

- Pinch salt

- 1 teaspoon pure vanilla extract

Directions:

1. Heat the almond milk, quinoa, coconut milk, maple syrup, salt, and vanilla over medium-high heat in a large saucepan.

2. Bring the quinoa mixture to a boil and then reduce the heat to low.

3. Simmer until the quinoa is tender, stirring frequently, about 20 minutes.

4. Remove the pudding from the heat.

5. Serve warm.

6. Flavor Boost: If you are a chocolate enthusiast, stir 1 tablespoon of good-quality unsweetened cocoa powder into the almond milk and coconut milk before you combine the liquids with the other ingredients in step 1. This way you can remove any lumps in the cocoa powder before you add the quinoa. Increase the maple syrup to ¾ cup to offset the bitterness of the powder.

Nutrition: Calories: 249 Total Fat: 6g Protein: 6g Cholesterol: 0mg Sodium: 161mg Carbohydrates: 42g Fiber: 3g

35. Stuffed Pears with Hazelnuts

Preparation Time: 5 minutes

Cooking Time: 20 minutes

Servings: 4

Ingredients:

- 1 tablespoon butter

- 2 ripe pears, cored and hollowed out with a spoon

- ½ cup water

- 8 tablespoons goat cheese

- 2 tablespoons honey

- ¼ cup roughly chopped hazelnuts

Directions:

1. Preheat the oven to 350°f.

2. Melt the butter using a skillet on a medium heat.

3. Place the pears in the skillet, skin-side up, and lightly brown them, about 2 minutes.

4. Place the pears in an 8-by-8-inch square baking dish, hollow-side up, and pour water into the baking dish, make sure not to get any in the hollow part of the pears.

5. Roast the pears until softened, about 10 minutes. Remove the pears from the oven.

6. Using a small bowl, mix goat cheese, honey, and hazelnuts.

7. Divide the goat cheese mixture evenly between the pear halves and put them back in the oven for 5 minutes. Serve warm.

Nutrition: Calories: 185 Total Fat: 9g Protein: 4g Cholesterol: 14mg Sodium: 75mg Carbohydrates: 26g Fiber: 4g

CHAPTER 7:

JUICES AND SMOOTHIES RECIPES

36. Healthy Purple Smoothie

Preparation Time: 3 minutes

Cooking Time: 0 minutes

Servings: 2

Ingredients:

- 2-3 frozen broccoli florets
- 1 cup water
- 1/2 avocado, peeled and chopped
- 3 plums, chopped

- 1 cup blueberries

Directions:

1. Combine all ingredients in a high-speed blender and blend until smooth.

Nutrition: Calories: 45 Carbohydrates: 3g Total fat: 2g Protein: 1g

37. Mom's Favourite Kale Smoothie

Preparation Time: 3 minutes

Cooking Time: 0 minutes

Servings: 2

Ingredients:

- 2-3 ice cubes
- 1½ cup orange juice
- 1 green small apple, cut
- ½ cucumber, chopped
- 2-3 leaves kale
- ½ cup raspberries

Directions:

1. Combine all ingredients in a high-speed blender and blend until smooth.

Nutrition: Calories: 51 Carbohydrates: 0g Total fat: 0g Protein: 0g

38. Creamy Green Smoothie

Preparation Time: 3 minutes

Cooking Time: 0 minutes

Servings: 2

Ingredients:

- 1 frozen banana
- 1 cup coconut milk
- 1 small pear, chopped
- 1 cup baby spinach
- 1 tsp. vanilla extract

Directions:

1. Combine all ingredients in a high-speed blender and blend until smooth.

Nutrition: Calories: 301 Carbohydrates: 21g Total fat: 9g Protein: 29g

39. Strawberry and Arugula Smoothie

Preparation Time: 3 minutes

Cooking Time: 0 minutes

Servings: 2

Ingredients:

- 2 cups frozen strawberries
- 1 cup unsweetened almond milk
- 10-12 arugula leaves
- 1/2 tsp. ground cinnamon

Directions:

1. Combine ice, almond milk, strawberries, arugula, and cinnamon in a high-speed blender. Blend until smooth and serve.

Nutrition: Calories: 2 Carbohydrates: 0g Total fat: 0g Protein: 0g

40. Emma's Amazing Smoothie

Preparation Time: 3 minutes

Cooking Time: 0 minutes

Servings: 2

Ingredients:

- 1 frozen banana, chopped
- 1 cup orange juice
- 1 large nectarine, sliced
- 1/2 zucchini, peeled and chopped
- 2-3 dates, pitted

Directions:

1. Combine all ingredients in a high-speed blender and blend until smooth.

Nutrition: Calories: 2 Carbohydrates: 0g Total fat: 0g Protein: 0g

41. Good-To-Go Morning Smoothie

Preparation Time: 3 minutes

Cooking Time: 0 minutes

Servings: 2

Ingredients:

- 1 cup frozen strawberries
- 1 cup apple juice
- 1 banana, chopped
- 1 cup raw asparagus, chopped
- 1 tbsp. ground flaxseed

Directions:

1. Combine all ingredients in a high-speed blender and blend until smooth.

Nutrition: Calories: 200 Carbohydrates: 25g Total fat: 0g Protein: 2g

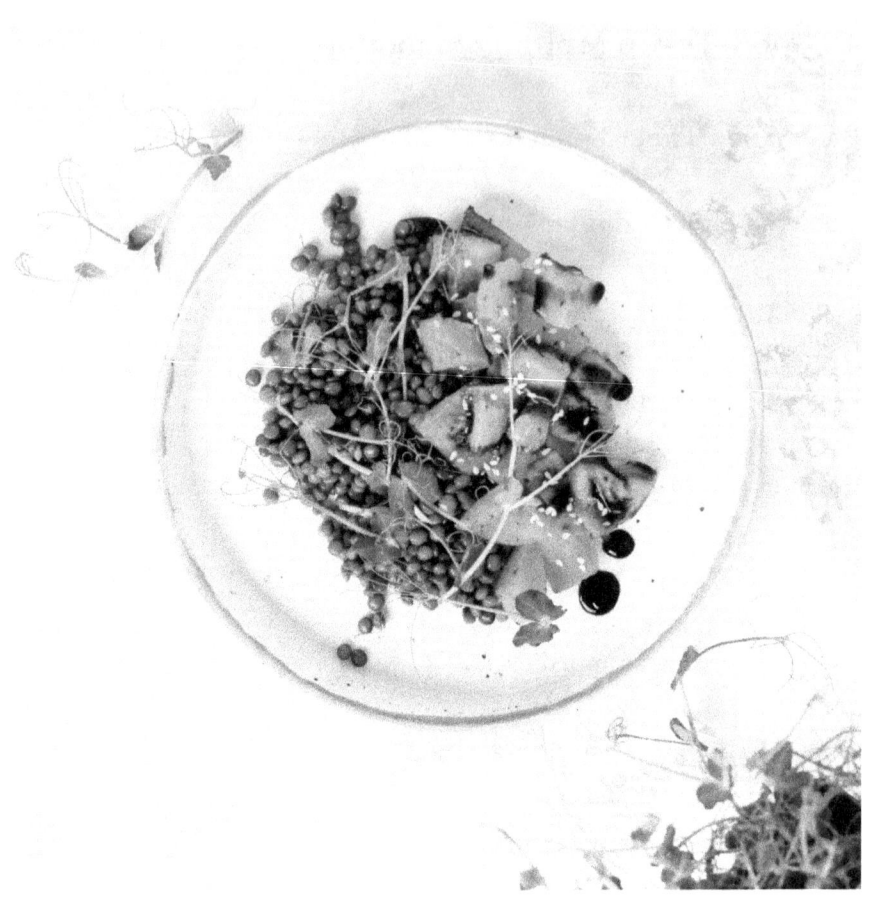

CHAPTER 8:

OTHER RECIPES

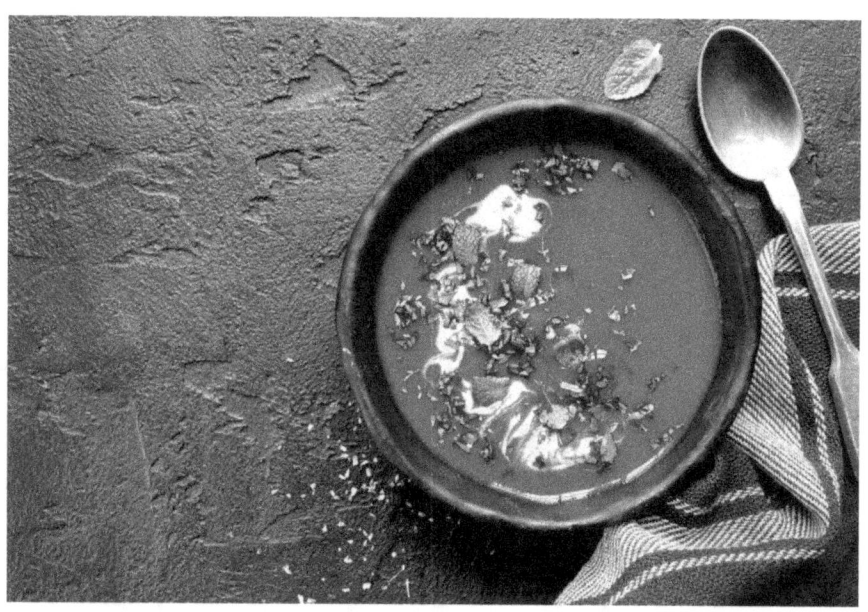

42. Spinach & orange salad

Preparation Time: 15 minutes

Cooking Time: 0 minutes

Servings: 6

Ingredients

- ¼ -⅓ cup vegan dressing
- 3 oranges, medium, peeled, seeded & sectioned
- ¾ lb. spinach, fresh & torn
- 1 red onion, medium, sliced & separated into rings

Directions:

1. Toss everything together and serve with dressing.

Nutrition: Calories: 100 Fat: 2 g Carbs: 12 g Protein: 5 g

43. Lime-macerated mangos

Preparation Time: 10 minutes

Cooking Time: 0 minutes

Servings: 5

Ingredients:

- 3 ripe mangos
- 1/3 cup light brown sugar
- 2 tablespoons fresh lime juice
- 1/2 cup dry white wine
- Fresh mint sprigs

Directions

1. Peel, pit, and cut the mangos into 1/2-inch dice. Layer the diced mango in a large bowl, sprinkling each layer with about 1 tablespoon of the sugar. Cover with plastic wrap and refrigerate for 2 hours.

2. Pour in the lime juice and wine, mixing gently to combine with the mango. Cover and refrigerate for 4 hours.

3. About 30 minutes before serving time, bring the fruit to room temperature. To serve, spoon the mango and the liquid into serving glasses and garnish with mint.

Nutrition: Calories: 150 Fat: 2g Carbs: 16 g Protein: 8 g

44. Raspberry chia pudding

Preparation Time: 10 minutes

Cooking Time: 0 minutes

Servings: 2

Ingredients

- 4 tablespoons chia seeds
- 1 cup coconut milk
- ½ cup raspberries

Directions:

1. Add raspberry and coconut milk in a blender and blend until smooth.
2. Pour mixture into the Mason jar.
3. Add chia seeds in a jar and stir well.
4. Close the jar tightly with lid and shake well.
5. Place in the refrigerator for 3 hours.
6. Serve chilled and enjoy.

Nutrition: Calories: 140 Fat: 5 g Carbs: 20 g Protein: 8 g

45. Lemon Mousse

Preparation Time: 10 minutes + 2 hours Cooking Time: 0 minutes

Servings: 2

Ingredients

- 14 oz. coconut milk
- 12 drops liquid stevia
- ½ tsp. lemon extract
- ¼ tsp. turmeric

Directions

1. Refrigerate a 1 can coconut milk overnight. Scoop out thick cream into a mixing bowl.
2. Add remaining ingredients to the bowl and whip using a hand mixer until smooth.
3. Transfer mousse mixture to a zip-lock bag and pipe into small serving glasses. Place in refrigerator.
4. Serve chilled and enjoy.

Nutrition: Calories: 200 Fat: 6 g Carbs: 28 g Protein: 8 g

46. Banana Mango Ice Cream

Preparation Time: 30 Minutes Cook Time: 0 Minutes

Servings: 2

Ingredients:

- 1 banana, peeled and sliced
- 2 ripe mangos with the skin removed, and the flesh cubed
- 3 tablespoons almond or cashew milk, chilled

Directions:

1. Lay out the banana and mango slices on a baking sheet lined with parchment paper and place them in the freezer.
2. Once they are frozen solid, remove the fruit and place it in the food processor.
3. Add the cold milk and process until smooth, about three to four minutes.
4. Taste and add sweetener as needed.
5. Serve immediately.

Nutrition: Calories 306 Fat 6.8g Carbohydrate 65.1g Protein 3.9g

47. Raspberry Chia Pudding Shots

Preparation Time: 1 hour Cook Time: 15 Minutes

Servings: 2

Ingredients:

- ¼ cup chia seeds
- ½ cup raspberries
- ½ cup coconut milk
- ¼ cup almond milk
- 1 Tbsps. cacao powder
- 1 Tbsps. stevia

Directions:

1. Combine all ingredients except raspberries in a jar.
2. Let sit for 2-3 minutes and transfer to shot glasses.
3. Refrigerate 1 hour or overnight to serve as breakfast.
4. Serve with fresh raspberries.

Nutrition: Calories 246 Fat 23.1g Carbohydrate 13.6g Protein 3.6g

48. Sautéed Bosc Pears with Walnuts

Preparation Time: 15 Minutes

Cook Time: 16 Minutes

Servings: 6

Ingredients:

- 2 Tbsps. salted butter
- ¼ tsp. cinnamon
- ¼ tsp. nutmeg, ground
- 6 Bosc pears, peeled, quartered
- 1 Tbsps. lemon juice
- ½ cup walnuts, chopped, toasted

Directions:

1. Melt butter in a skillet, add spices, and cook for 30 seconds.
2. Add pears and cook for 15 minutes. Stir in lemon juice.
3. Serve topped with walnuts.

Nutrition: Calories 221 Fat 10.3g Carbohydrate 33g Protein 3.3g

49. Mango & Papaya After-Chop

Preparation Time: 25 Minutes

Cook Time: 0 Minutes

Servings: 1

Ingredients:

- ¼ of papaya, chopped
- 1 mango, chopped
- 1 Tbsps. coconut milk
- ½ tsp. maple syrup
- 1 Tbsps. peanuts, chopped

Directions:

1. Cut open the papaya. Scoop out the seeds, chop.
2. Peel the mango. Slice the fruit from the pit, chop.
3. Put the fruit in a bowl. Add remaining ingredients. Stir to coat.

Nutrition: Calories 330 Fat 9.6g Carbohydrate 63.4g Protein 5.8g

50. Greek-style garbanzo beans

Preparation Time: 8 hours 5 minutes

Cook Time: 10 hours

Servings: 10

Ingredients:

- 12 ounces garbanzo beans
- 14 oz. tomatoes with juice, chopped
- 2 stalks celery, diced
- 1 onion, diced
- 4 garlic cloves, minced
- ¼ tsp. Salt

Directions:

1. Soak beans in water for 8 hours.
2. Combine drained beans with the remaining ingredients. Stir and pour water to cover.
3. Cook for 10 hours on low. Season with salt and serve.

Nutrition: Calories 138 Fat 2.2g Carbohydrate 23.7g Protein 7.1g

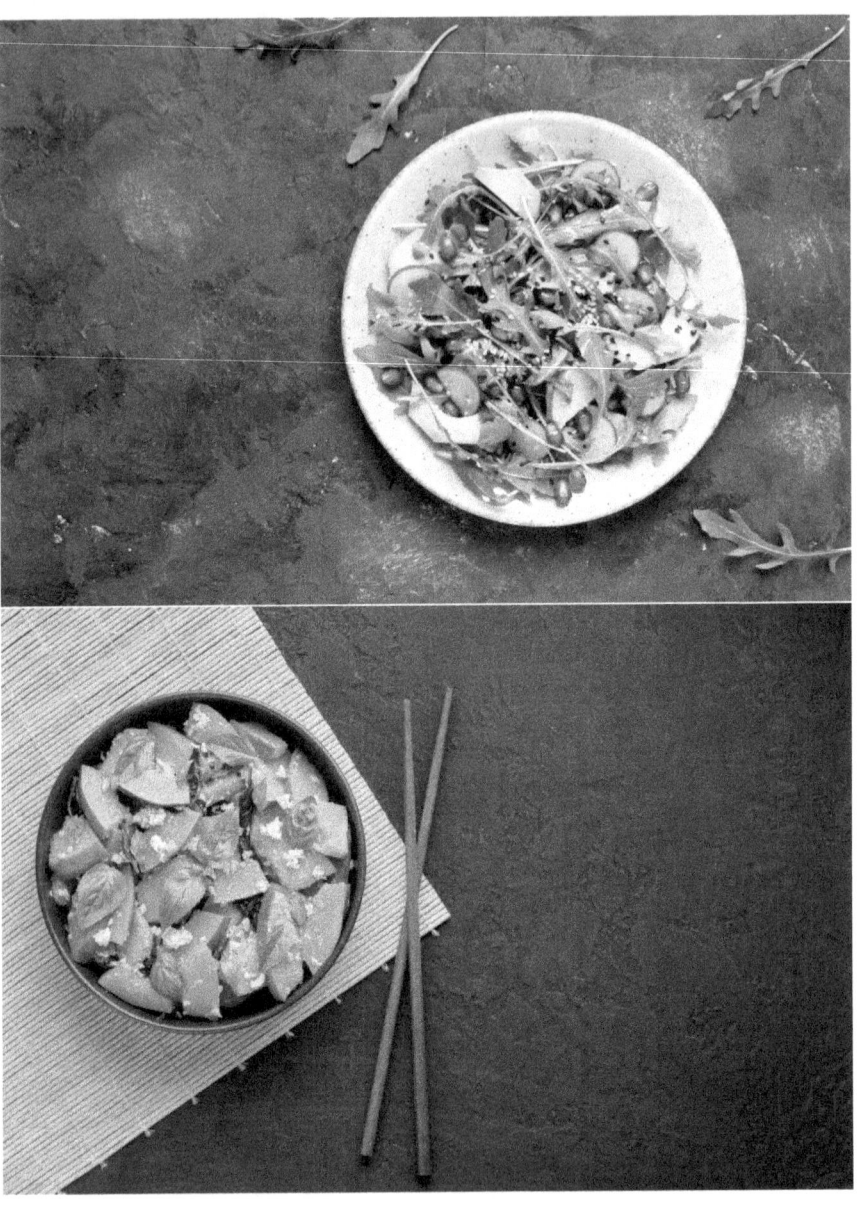

CONCLUSION

Well done! Thank you for reaching the end of this book, The Complete Vegetarian Cookbook.

Hopefully, this book has helped you understand that making vegetarian recipes and diet easier can improve your life, not only by improving your health and helping you lose weight, but also by saving you money and time.

Remember that vegetarianism is a choice, not a religion.

Be flexible when it comes to your diet and enjoy new tastes and experiences.

Don't be afraid of meat substitutes, but experiment with using them sparingly. There is no need to completely replace meat with fake meat products like tofu or processed soy-based vegetarian burgers and hot dogs. Not only are they expensive, but fake meats contain artificial ingredients that may or may not be healthy for you.

Also, if you are not used to eating a vegetarian diet, start with a few vegetarian meals and snacks during the week, and see how you feel.

You can always add more vegetarian meals to your diet later. It is better to be even slightly vegetarians than completely non-vegetarian.

The best tip I can give you about making vegetarian recipes is to experiment and have fun!

Here are some more tips to help you with your vegetarian diet:

1. Remember that vegetarianism is not a destination, it is a journey.

2. A vegetarian diet is plant-based. This means that you should try to eat more plants and less animal products. You should also be careful not to replace whole foods with their processed counterparts, such as replacing whole foods such as fruits and vegetables with fruit juice and pasta sauce.

3. Try to avoid processed food whenever possible, while still maintaining your balanced diet and nutrients that you need for your health. An easier way of doing this will be to make your own food when

possible and try to avoid packaged, pre-prepared foods at the grocery store.

4. Avoid processed food products that contain artificial ingredients, such as sweeteners, colors, and flavors.

5. Avoid highly processed meat substitutes. Remember to use meat substitutes in moderation or as an occasional treat.

6. If you choose to eat meat substitutes such as tofu, be sure to thoroughly cook it and try different ways of preparing it

7. You may need to gradually introduce your family and friends to your new eating habits. Don't expect everyone to support you or enjoy the same things you do when it comes to vegetarian recipes. As long as you are happy with your food choices, that is the most important thing – even if it means making some changes at home!

When you are having a hard time, always remember this: You can always choose to stop being a vegetarian.

You can simply start eating meat again if you are struggling with your new diet.

Remember that it is okay to be a part-time vegetarian, but if you find that you cannot maintain the lifestyle or are unhappy with your choice, it is always better to go back to eating a non-veg diet.

There is no shame in making changes to your vegetarian recipe routine if you need to, and you will not shame yourself for deciding that a strict vegetarian diet does not work for you.

I know that there are many books and choosing my book is amazing. I am thankful that you stopped and took the time to decide. You made a great decision, and I am sure that you enjoyed it.

I will be even happier if you will add some comments. Feedbacks helped by growing, and they still do. They help me to choose better content and new ideas. So, maybe your feedback can trigger an idea for my next book. Thank you again for downloading this book!

I hope you enjoyed reading my book!

www.ingramcontent.com/pod-product-compliance
Lightning Source LLC
Chambersburg PA
CBHW070934080526
44589CB00013B/1507